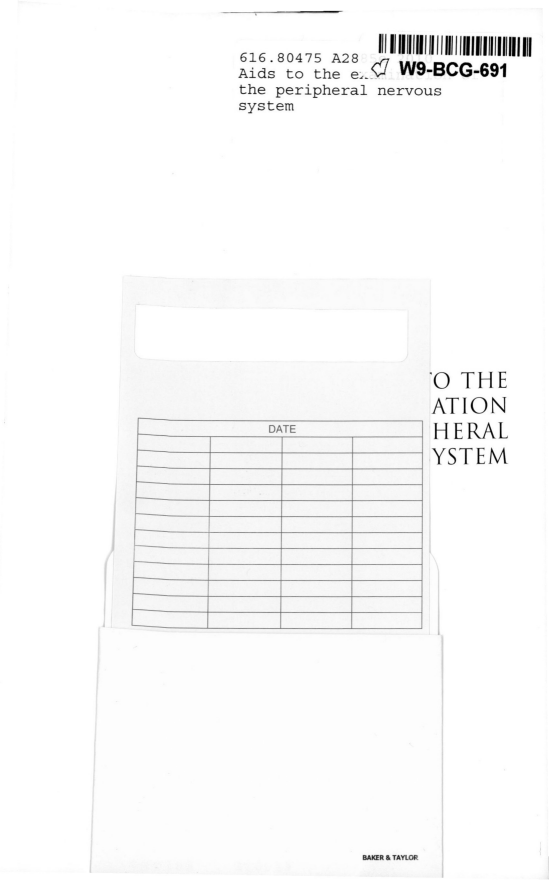

O THE
ATION
HERAL
YSTEM

	DATE		

For Elsevier
Publisher: Timothy Horne
Development Editor: Sheila Black
Project Manager: Glenys Norquay
Designer: Stewart Larking
Illustration Manager: Bruce Hogarth
Illustrator: Antbits

FIFTH EDITION

AIDS TO THE EXAMINATION OF THE PERIPHERAL NERVOUS SYSTEM

Edinburgh   London   New York   Oxford
Philadelphia   St Louis   Sydney   Toronto 2010

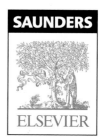

SAUNDERS
ELSEVIER

An imprint of Elsevier Limited

ISBN 978-0-7020-3447-3
   Reprinted 2011, 2012, 2013 (twice)

British Library Cataloguing in Publication Data
A catalogue record for this book is available from the British Library

Library of Congress Cataloging in Publication Data
A catalog record for this book is available from the Library of Congress

Notices
Knowledge and best practice in this field are constantly changing. As new research and
experience broaden our understanding, changes in research methods, professional
practices, or medical treatment may become necessary.

Practitioners and researchers must always rely on their own experience and knowledge
in evaluating and using any information, methods, compounds, or experiments
described herein. In using such information or methods they should be mindful of their
own safety and the safety of others, including parties for whom they have a
professional responsibility.

To the fullest extent of the law, neither the Publisher nor the authors, contributors, or
editors, assume any liability for any injury and/or damage to persons or property as a
matter of products liability, negligence or otherwise, or from any use or operation of
any methods, products, instructions, or ideas contained in the material herein.

ELSEVIER   your source for books,
journals and multimedia
in the health sciences
www.elsevierhealth.com

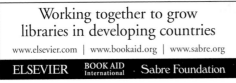

Working together to grow
libraries in developing countries

www.elsevier.com | www.bookaid.org | www.sabre.org

ELSEVIER   BOOK AID International · Sabre Foundation

The
publisher's
policy is to use
paper manufactured
from sustainable forests

Printed in China

In 1940 Dr George Riddoch was Consultant Neurologist to the Army. He realised the necessity of providing centres to deal with peripheral nerve injuries during the war. In collaboration with Professor J. R. Learmonth, Professor of Surgery at the University of Edinburgh, peripheral nerve injury centres were established at the neurosurgical units at Gogarburn near Edinburgh and at Killearn near Glasgow. Professor Learmonth suggested an illustrated guide on peripheral nerve injuries for the use of surgeons working in general hospitals. In collaboration with Dr Ritchie Russell, a few photographs demonstrating the testing of individual muscles were taken in 1941. Dr Ritchie Russell returned to Oxford in 1942 and was replaced by Dr M. J. McArdle as Neurologist to Scottish Command. The photographs were completed by Dr McArdle at Gogarburn with the help of the Department of Medical Illustration at the University of Edinburgh. About twenty copies in loose-leaf format were circulated to surgeons in Scotland.

In 1942 Professor Learmonth and Dr Riddoch added the diagrams illustrating the innervation of muscles by various peripheral nerves (modified from Pitres J-A and Testut L. *Les Nerfs en Schémas*, Doin, Paris, 1925) and also the diagrams of cutaneous sensory distributions and dermatomes. This was first published by the Medical Research Council in 1942 as *Aids to the Investigation of Peripheral Nerve Injuries* (War Memorandum No. 7) and revised in 1943. It became a standard work and over the next thirty years many thousands of copies were printed.

It was thoroughly revised between 1972 and 1975 with new photographs and many new diagrams and was republished under the title *Aids to the Examination of the Peripheral Nervous System* (Memorandum No. 45), reflecting the wide use made of this booklet by students and practitioners and its more extensive use in clinical neurology, which was rather different from the wartime emphasis on nerve injuries.

In 1984 the Medical Research Council transferred responsibility for this publication to the Guarantors of *Brain*, for whom a new edition was prepared. Modifications were made to some of the diagrams and a new diagram of the lumbosacral plexus was included.

Most of the photographs for the 1943, 1975 and 1986 editions show Dr McArdle, who died in 1989, as the examining physician. A new set of colour photographs was prepared for the Fourth Edition; the diagrams of the brachial plexus and lumbosacral plexus were retained, but all the other diagrams were redrawn. The Introduction for the Fifth Edition has been revised and new diagrams of the cutaneous distribution of the trigeminal nerve added. There have been some minor modifications to existing figures.

M.D. O'Brien
for The Guarantors of *Brain*

MRC Nerve injuries committee 1942–1943

Brigadier G. Riddoch, MD, FRCP (*Chairman*)
Brigadier W. Rowley Bristow, MB, FRCS
G. L. Brown, MSc, MB (*1942*)
Brigadier H. W. B. Cairns, DM, FRCS
E. A. Carmichael, CBE, MB, FRCP
Surgeon Captain M. Critchley, MD, FRCP, RNVR
J. G. Greenfield, MD, FRCP
Professor J. R. Learmonth, CBE, ChM, FRCSE
Professor H. Platt, MD, FRCS
Professor H. J. Seddon, DM, FRCS (*1942*)
Air Commodore C. P. Symonds, MD, FRCP
J. Z. Young, MA
F. J. C. Herrald, MB, MRCPE (*Secretary*)

MRC Revision subcommittee 1972–1975

Sir Herbert Seddon, CMG, DM, FRCS (*Chairman until October 1973*)
Professor J. N. Walton, TD, MD, DSC, FRCP (*Chairman from October 1973*)
Professor R. W. Gilliatt, DM, FRCP
M. J. F. McArdle, MB, FRCP
M. D. O'Brien, MD, MRCP
Professor P. K. Thomas, DSC, MD, FRCP
R. G. Willison, DM, FRCPE

Editorial Committee for the Guarantors of *Brain* 1984–1986

Sir John Walton, TD, MD, DSC, FRCP (*Chairman*)
Professor R. W. Gilliatt, DM, FRCP
M. Hutchinson, MB, BDS
M. J. F. McArdle, MB, FRCP
M. D. O'Brien, MD, FRCP
Professor P. K. Thomas, DSC, MD, FRCP
R. G. Willison, DM, FRCPE

4th edition prepared for the Guarantors of *Brain* 1999–2000

5th edition prepared for the Guarantors of *Brain* 2009–2010

M. D. O'Brien, MD, FRCP

ACKNOWLEDGEMENTS

The Guarantors of *Brain* are very grateful to:

Patricia Archer PhD for the drawings of the brachial plexus and lumbosacral plexus
Ralph Hutchings for the photography
Paul Richardson and **Richard Tibbitts** for the artwork and diagrams
Michael Hutchinson MB BDS for advice on the neuro-anatomy
Sarah Keer-Keer (Harcourt Publishers) for her help and encouragement.

CONTENTS

This atlas is intended as a guide to the examination of patients with lesions of peripheral nerves or nerve roots.

Examination should, if possible, be conducted in a warm and quiet room where patient and examiner will be free from distraction. Most patients will be unfamiliar with the procedures in a neurological examination, so that the nature and object of the tests should be explained in some detail to secure their interest and co-operation.

MOTOR TESTING

Inspection: look for abnormal posture, wasting and fasciculation with the limb at rest.
Tone: in adults, the assessment of tone is only useful for upper motor neuron lesions.
Power: muscle power is assessed by testing the strength of movement at a single joint, which is usually achieved by more than one muscle acting in different ways, and these may have different spinal root and peripheral nerve supplies.

A muscle may act as a *prime mover*, as a *fixator*, as an *antagonist*, or as a *synergist*. Thus, flexor carpi ulnaris acts as a *prime mover* when it flexes and adducts the wrist; as a *fixator* when it immobilises the pisiform bone during contraction of the adductor digiti minimi; as an *antagonist* when it resists extension of the wrist; and as a *synergist* when the digits, but not the wrists, are extended.

CHOICE OF MOVEMENT

Ideally, movements should be chosen which help to differentiate upper from lower motor neuron lesions and be innervated by a single spinal root and peripheral nerve; and in peripheral nerve lesions, to identify the affected nerve and the site of the lesion. Therefore, preference should be given to muscles which have a single root innervation and preferably an easily elicitable reflex, a single peripheral nerve innervation, be the main or only muscle effecting the movement and one that can be seen and felt. This is not often possible, especially in the lower limb. The table on p 64 lists the commonly tested movements, indicates whether they are preferentially affected in upper motor neuron lesions, and gives their principal root supply, relevant reflex, if there is one, peripheral nerve and main effector muscle.

TECHNIQUE

When testing a movement, the limb should be firmly supported proximal to the relevant joint, so that the test is confined to the chosen muscle group and does not require the patient to fix the limb proximally by muscle contraction. In this book, this principle is illustrated in Figs 12, 18, 28B, 31 and many others. In some illustrations, the examiner's supporting hand has been omitted for clarity (for example Figs 30, 34, 48 and 53). The amount of leverage applied should be such that a patient with normal strength is evenly matched with the examiner, so that minimal weakness is more easily appreciated (for example Figs 21, 70). However, the same technique should be used for all patients, so that the examiner can acquire experience of the variability in strength of different subjects. Optimal techniques are illustrated in the figures.

Muscle power may be recorded using the Medical Research Council scale, but this is not a linear scale and subdivisions of grade 4 are often necessary. Grades 4−, 4 and 4+ may be used to indicate movement against slight, moderate and strong resistance respectively.

MRC SCALE FOR MUSCLE STRENGTH

0	No contraction
1	Flicker or trace of contraction
2	Full range of active movement, with gravity eliminated
3	Active movement against gravity
4	Active movement against gravity and resistance
5	Normal power

Muscles have been arranged in the order of the origin of their motor supply from nerve trunks, which is convenient in many examinations. The usual nerve supply to each muscle is stated in the captions, and the spinal segments from which it is derived, the more important of these are printed in heavy type. The peripheral nerve diagrams show the usual order of innervation as a guide to the location of a lesion. Tables showing limb muscles arranged according to their supply by individual nerve roots and peripheral nerves are to be found on pp 62–63.

SENSORY TESTING

Asking the patient to outline the area of sensory abnormality can be a useful guide to the detailed examination. If this clearly indicates the distribution of a peripheral nerve, for example the lateral cutaneous nerve of the thigh (meralgia paraesthetica, Fig. 59), the area can be mapped to light touch, tested with cotton wool or a light finger touch, and to pain using a clean pin (not a needle which is designed to cut the skin). In both cases, work from the insensitive towards an area of normal sensation. If the area of sensory abnormality is hypersensitive (hyperpathia), the direction is reversed.

Otherwise, it may be helpful to divide sensory testing into those modalities which travel in the ipsilateral posterior columns of the spinal cord (light touch, vibration and joint position sense) and those that travel in the crossed spinothalamic tracts (pain and temperature appreciation). Appreciation of vibration, a repetitive touch/pressure stimulus, is a sensitive test for demyelinating peripheral neuropathies. Two point discrimination is a sensitive and quantifiable test of light touch, but it is only reliable on the face and finger tips. Always start with a stimulus at or below the normal threshold and coarsen the stimulus as required.

There is considerable overlap in the area of skin (dermatome) supplied by consecutive nerve roots, so that section of a single root may result in a very small area of sensory impairment. Conversely, the rash of herpes zoster may be quite extensive, because it affects the whole area which has any supply from the affected root. The dermatome illustrations in Figs 88–94 are a compromise. The heavier axial lines, which separate non-consecutive dermatomes, are more reliable as boundaries. The area of impairment with a peripheral nerve lesion is more reliable and consistent than that from a nerve root lesion. The areas shown in the diagrams are the usual ones. Some nerves show considerable variation between patients (see Figs 25 and 59) and others are much more consistent: for example the ulnar nerve reliably splits at least part of the ring finger (see Fig. 46).

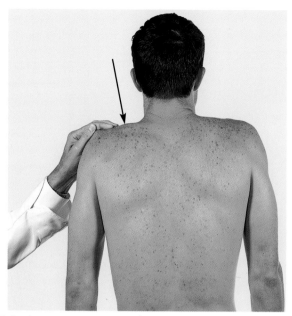

Fig. 1 Trapezius (Spinal accessory nerve and C3, C4)
The patient is elevating the shoulder against resistance.
Arrow: the thick upper part of the muscle can be seen and felt.

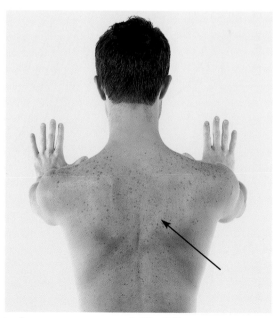

Fig. 2 Trapezius (Spinal accessory nerve and C3, C4)
The patient is pushing the palms of the hands hard against a wall with the elbows fully
extended. *Arrow*: the lower fibres of trapezius can be seen and felt.

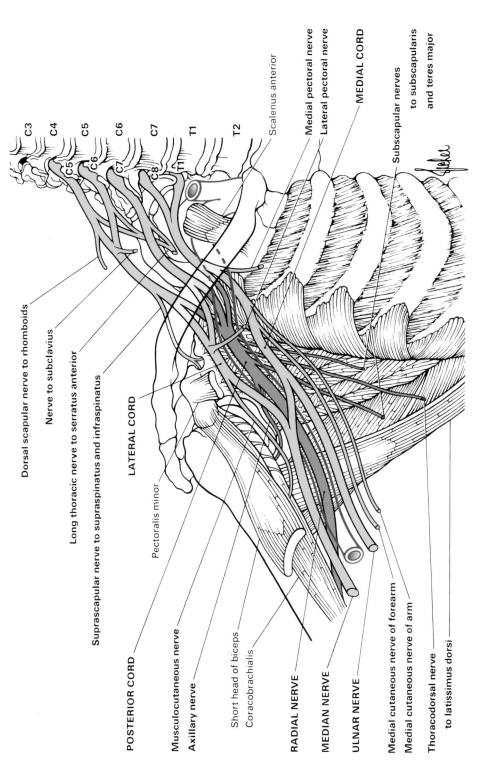

Fig. 3 Diagram of the brachial plexus, its branches and the muscles which they supply.

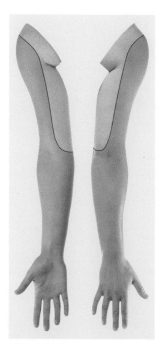

Fig. 4 The approximate area within which sensory changes may be found in complete lesions of the brachial plexus (C5, C6, C7, C8, T1).

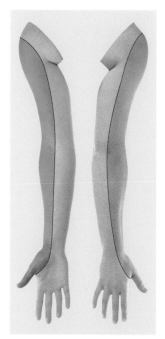

Fig. 5 The approximate area within which sensory changes may be found in lesions of the upper roots (C5, C6) of the brachial plexus.

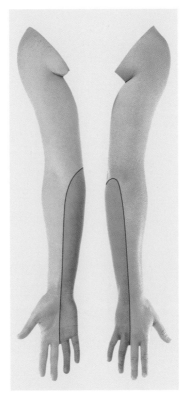

Fig. 6 The approximate area within which sensory changes may be found in lesions of the lower roots (C8, T1) of the brachial plexus.

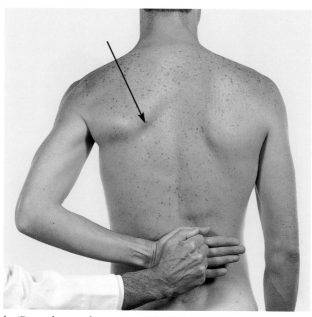

Fig. 7 Rhomboids (Dorsal scapular nerve; C4, C5)
The patient is pressing the palm of his hand backwards against the examiner's hand.
Arrow: the muscle bellies can be felt and sometimes seen.

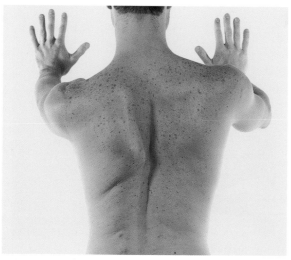

Fig. 8 Serratus Anterior (Long thoracic nerve; C5, C6, C7)
The patient is pushing against a wall. The left serratus anterior is paralysed and there is winging of the scapula.

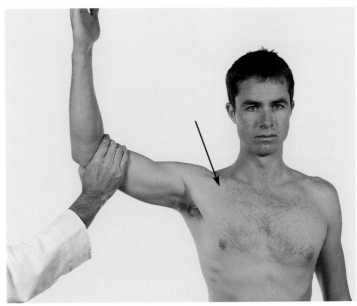

Fig. 9 Pectoralis Major: Clavicular Head (Lateral pectoral nerve; **C5**, **C6**)
The upper arm is above the horizontal and the patient is pushing forward against the examiner's hand. *Arrow:* the clavicular head of pectoralis major can be seen and felt.

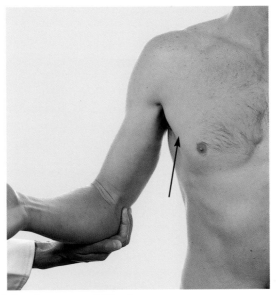

Fig. 10 Pectoralis Major: Sternocostal Head
(Lateral and medial pectoral nerves; C6, **C7**, C8)
The patient is adducting the upper arm against resistance.
Arrow: the sternocostal head can be seen and felt.

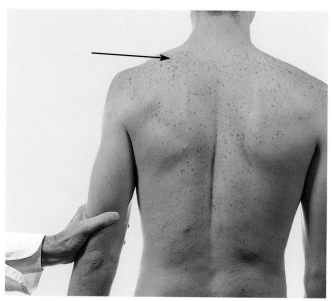

Fig. 11 Supraspinatus (Suprascapular nerve; C5, C6)
The patient is abducting the upper arm against resistance.
Arrow: the muscle belly can be felt and sometimes seen.

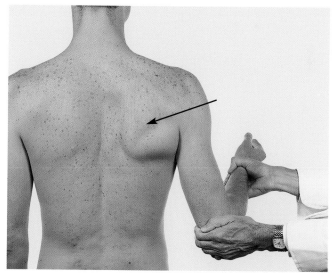

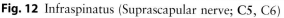

Fig. 12 Infraspinatus (Suprascapular nerve; C5, C6)
The patient is externally rotating the upper arm at the shoulder against resistance. The examiner's right hand is resisting the movement and supporting the forearm with the elbow at a right angle; his left hand is supporting the elbow and preventing abduction of the arm. *Arrow:* the muscle belly can be seen and felt.

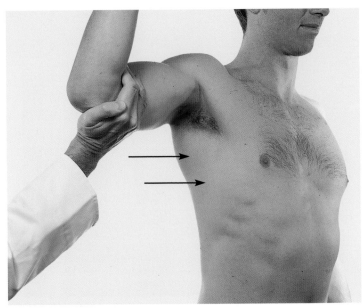

Fig. 13 Latissimus Dorsi (Thoracodorsal nerve; C6, **C7**, C8)
The upper arm is horizontal and the patient is adducting it against resistance. *Lower arrow:* the muscle belly can be seen and felt. The *upper arrow* points to teres major.

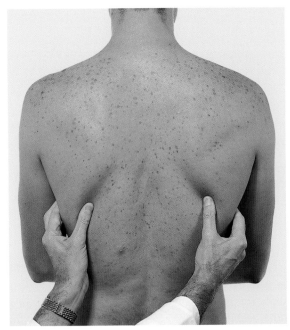

Fig. 14 Latissimus Dorsi (Thoracodorsal nerve; C6, **C7**, C8)
The muscle bellies can be felt to contract when the patient coughs.

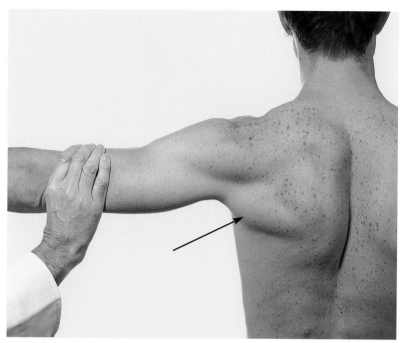

Fig. 15 Teres Major (Subscapular nerve; C5, C6, C7)
The patient is adducting the elevated upper arm against resistance.
Arrow: the muscle belly can be seen and felt.

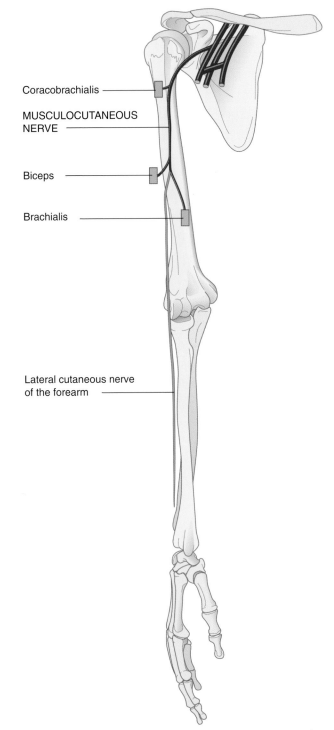

Coracobrachialis

MUSCULOCUTANEOUS
NERVE

Biceps

Brachialis

Lateral cutaneous nerve
of the forearm

Fig. 16 Diagram of the musculocutaneous nerve, its major cutaneous branch and the
muscles which it supplies.

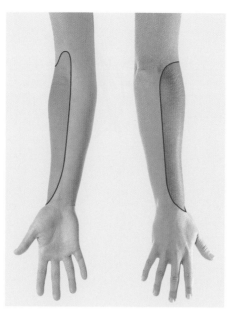

Fig. 17 The approximate area within which sensory changes may be found in lesions of the musculocutaneous nerve.
(The distribution of the lateral cutaneous nerve of the forearm.)

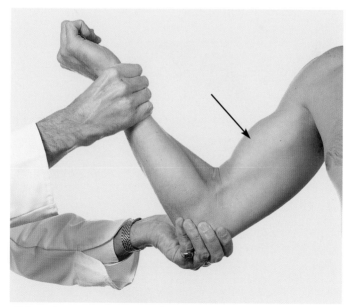

Fig. 18 Biceps (Musculocutaneous nerve; C5, C6)
The patient is flexing the supinated forearm against resistance.
Arrow: the muscle belly can be seen and felt.

AXILLARY NERVE

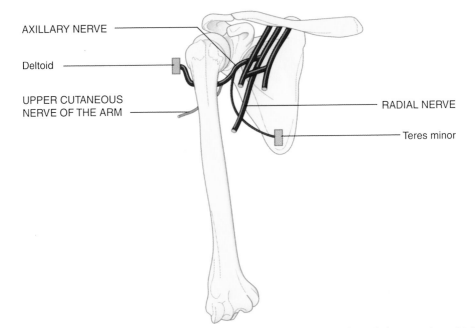

AXILLARY NERVE

Deltoid

UPPER CUTANEOUS
NERVE OF THE ARM

RADIAL NERVE

Teres minor

Fig. 19 Diagram of the axillary nerve, its major cutaneous branch and the muscles which it supplies.

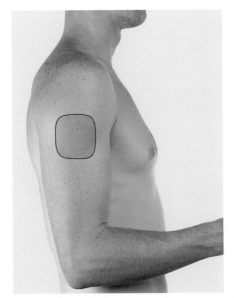

Fig. 20 The approximate area within which sensory changes may be found in lesions of the axillary nerve.

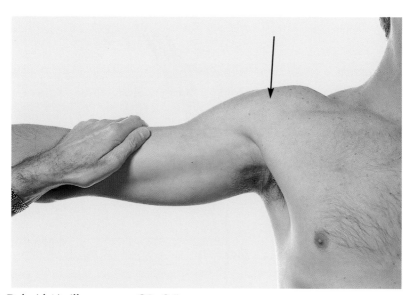

Fig. 21 Deltoid (Axillary nerve; C5, C6)
The patient is abducting the upper arm against resistance.
Arrow: the anterior and middle fibres of the muscle can be seen and felt.

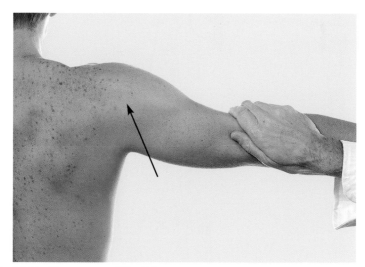

Fig. 22 Deltoid (Axillary nerve; C5, C6)
The patient is retracting the abducted upper arm against resistance.
Arrow: the posterior fibres of deltoid can be seen and felt.

RADIAL NERVE

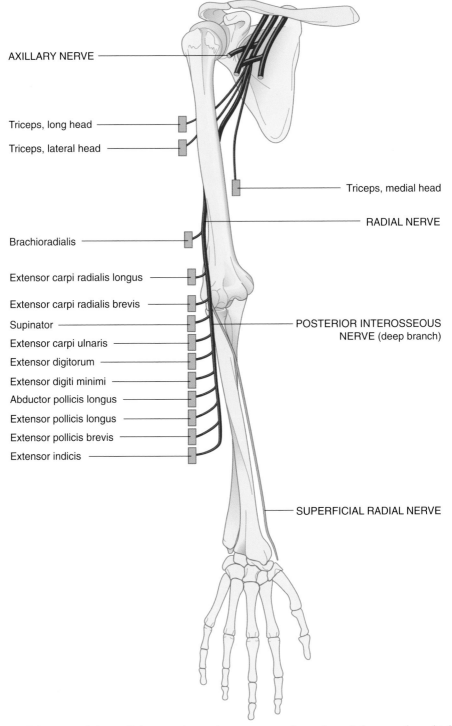

AXILLARY NERVE

Triceps, long head

Triceps, lateral head

Triceps, medial head

RADIAL NERVE

Brachioradialis

Extensor carpi radialis longus

Extensor carpi radialis brevis

Supinator

POSTERIOR INTEROSSEOUS
NERVE (deep branch)

Extensor carpi ulnaris

Extensor digitorum

Extensor digiti minimi

Abductor pollicis longus

Extensor pollicis longus

Extensor pollicis brevis

Extensor indicis

SUPERFICIAL RADIAL NERVE

Fig. 23 Diagram of the radial nerve, its major cutaneous branch and the muscles which it supplies.

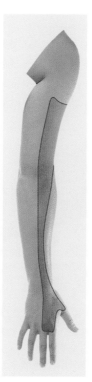

Fig. 24 The approximate area within which sensory changes may be found in high lesions of the radial nerve (above the origin of the posterior cutaneous nerves of the arm and forearm). The average area is usually considerably smaller, and absence of sensory changes has been recorded.

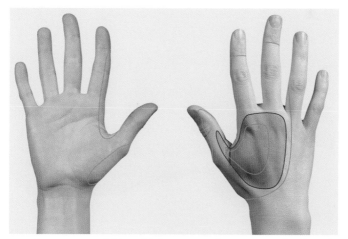

Fig. 25 The approximate area within which sensory changes may be found in lesions of the radial nerve above the elbow joint and below the origin of the posterior cutaneous nerve of the forearm. (The distribution of the superficial terminal branch of the radial nerve.) Usual area shaded, with dark blue line; light blue lines show small and large areas.

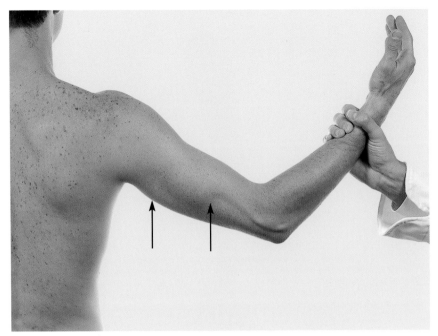

Fig. 26 Triceps (Radial nerve; C6, **C7**, C8)
The patient is extending the forearm at the elbow against resistance.
Arrows: the long and lateral heads of the muscle can be seen and felt.

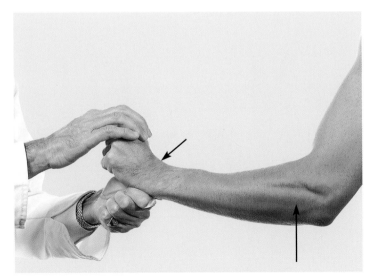

Fig. 27 Extensor Carpi Radialis Longus (Radial nerve; **C5, C6**)
The patient is extending and abducting the hand at the wrist against resistance.
Arrows: the muscle belly and tendon can be felt and usually seen.

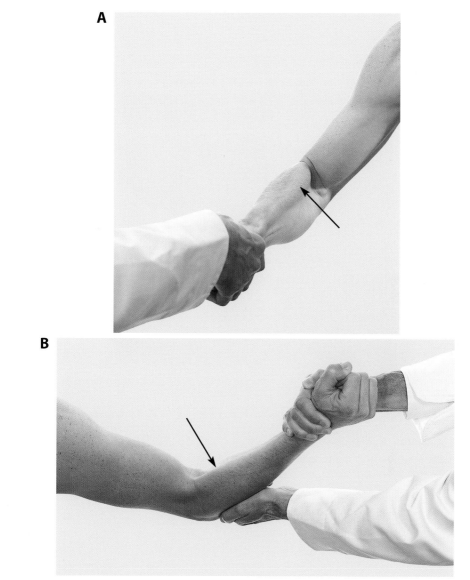

Fig. 28 Brachioradialis (Radial nerve; C5, C6)

The patient is flexing the forearm against resistance with the forearm midway between pronation and supination. *Arrow:* the muscle belly can be seen and felt.

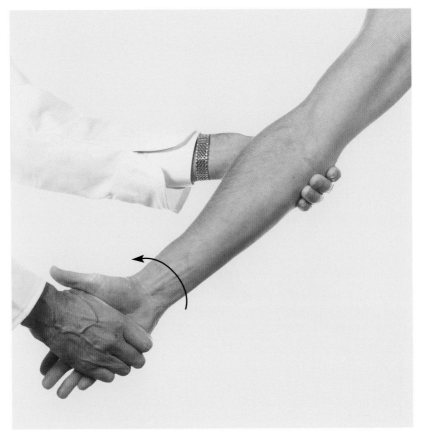

Fig. 29 Supinator (Radial nerve; C6, C7)
The patient is supinating the forearm against resistance with the forearm extended at the elbow.

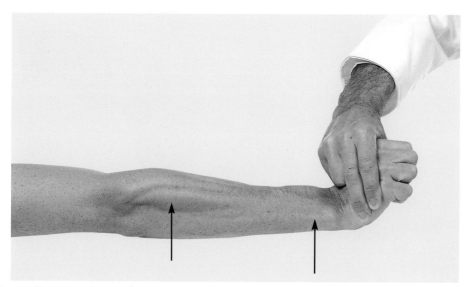

Fig. 30 Extensor Carpi Ulnaris (Posterior interosseous nerve; C7, C8)
The patient is extending and adducting the hand at the wrist against resistance.
Arrows: the muscle belly and the tendon can be seen and felt.

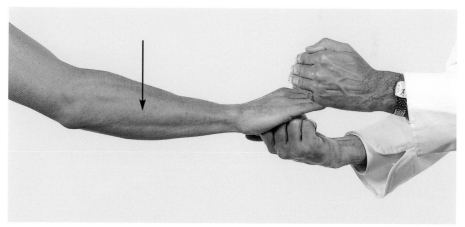

Fig. 31 Extensor Digitorum (Posterior interosseous nerve; C7, C8)
The patient's hand is firmly supported by the examiner's right hand. Extension at the
metacarpophalangeal joints is maintained against the resistance of the fingers of the
examiner's left hand. *Arrow:* the muscle belly can be seen and felt.

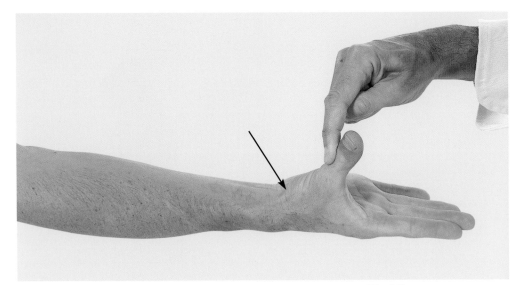

Fig. 32 Abductor Pollicis Longus (Posterior interosseous nerve; C7, C8)
The patient is abducting the thumb at the carpo-metacarpal joint in a plane at right angles to the palm. *Arrow:* the tendon can be seen and felt anterior and closely adjacent to the tendon of extensor pollicis brevis (**cf.** Fig. 34).

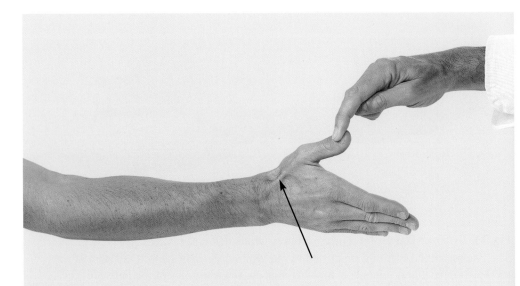

Fig. 33 Extensor Pollicis Longus (Posterior interosseous nerve; C7, C8)
The patient is extending the thumb at the interphalangeal joint against resistance.
Arrow: the tendon can be seen and felt.

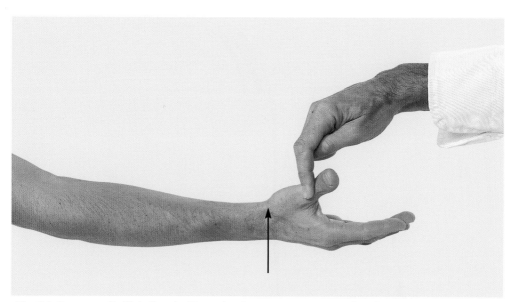

Fig. 34 Extensor Pollicis Brevis (Posterior interosseous nerve; **C7, C8**)
The patient is extending the thumb at the metacarpophalangeal joint against resistance.
Arrow: the tendon can be seen and felt (**cf.** Fig. 32).

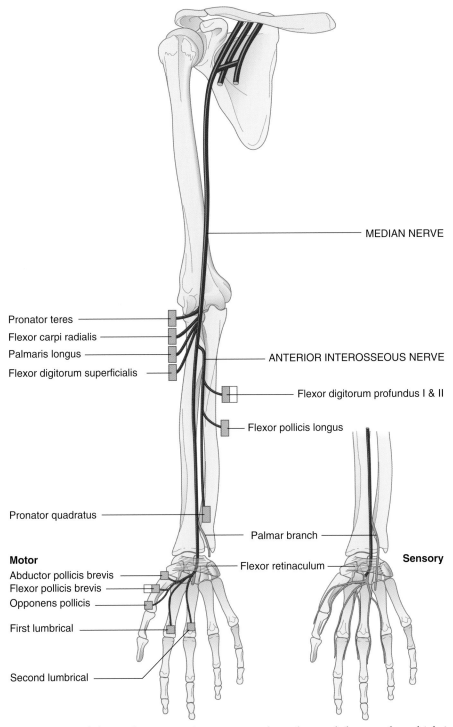

MEDIAN NERVE

Pronator teres

Flexor carpi radialis

Palmaris longus

Flexor digitorum superficialis

ANTERIOR INTEROSSEOUS NERVE

Flexor digitorum profundus I & II

Flexor pollicis longus

Pronator quadratus

Palmar branch

Motor

Abductor pollicis brevis

Flexor pollicis brevis

Opponens pollicis

First lumbrical

Second lumbrical

Flexor retinaculum

Sensory

Fig. 35 Diagram of the median nerve, its cutaneous branches and the muscles which it supplies. Note: the white rectangle signifies that the muscle indicated receives a part of its nerve supply from another peripheral nerve (**cf**. Figs 45, 57 and 58).

A

B

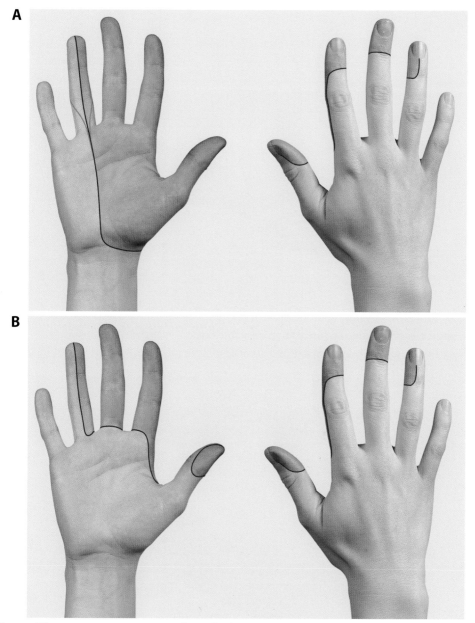

Fig. 36 The approximate areas within which sensory changes may be found in lesions of the median nerve in: **A** the forearm, **B** the carpal tunnel, note sparing of the palmar branch which does not go through the carpal tunnel.

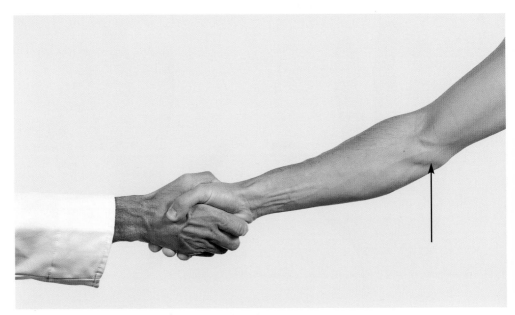

Fig. 37 Pronator Teres (Median nerve; C6, C7)
The patient is pronating the forearm against resistance.
Arrow: the muscle belly can be felt and sometime seen.

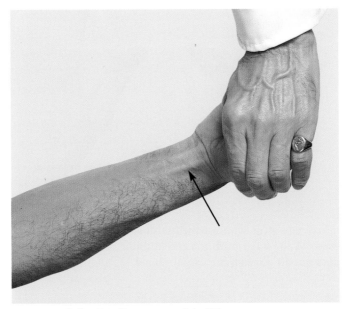

Fig. 38 Flexor Carpi Radialis (Median nerve; C6, C7)
The patient is flexing and abducting the hand at the wrist against resistance.
Arrow: the tendon can be seen and felt.

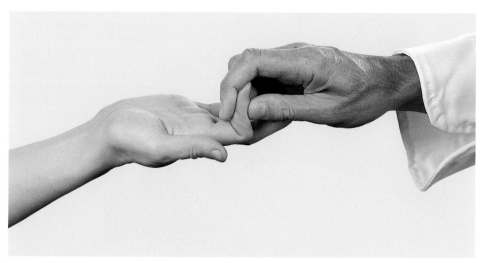

Fig. 39 Flexor Digitorum Superficialis (Median nerve; C7, **C8**, T1)
The patient is flexing the finger at the proximal interphalangeal joint against resistance with the proximal phalanx fixed. This test does not eliminate the possibility of flexion at the proximal interphalangeal joint being produced by flexor digitorum profundus.

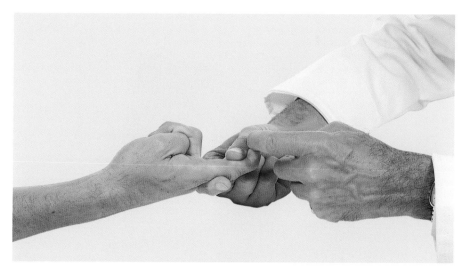

Fig. 40 Flexor Digitorum Profundus I and II (Anterior interosseous nerve; C7, C8)
The patient is flexing the distal phalanx of the index finger against resistance with the middle phalanx fixed.

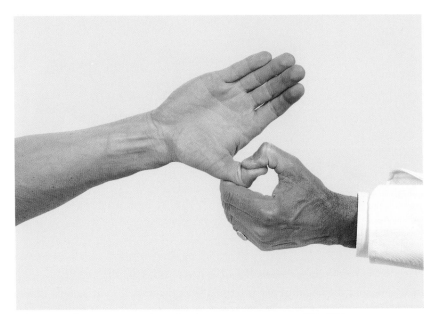

Fig. 41 Flexor Pollicis Longus (Anterior interosseous nerve; C7, **C8**)
The patient is flexing the distal phalanx of the thumb against resistance while the proximal phalanx is fixed.

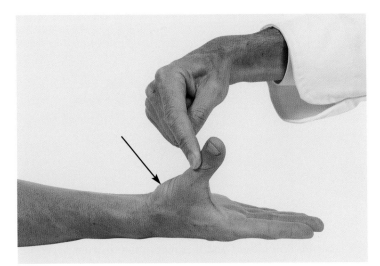

Fig. 42 Abductor Pollicis Brevis (Median nerve; C8, **T1**)
The patient is abducting the thumb at right angles to the palm against resistance.
Arrow: the muscle can be seen and felt.

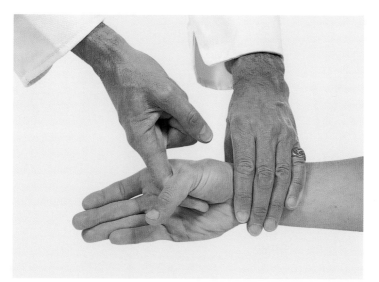

Fig. 43 Opponens Pollicis (Median nerve; C8, T1)
The patient is touching the base of the little finger with the thumb against resistance.

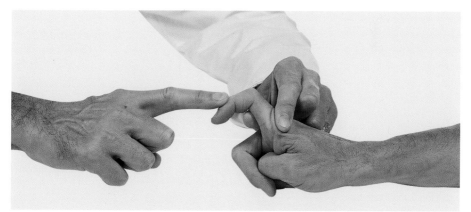

Fig. 44 1st Lumbrical-Interosseous Muscle (Median and ulnar nerves; C8, T1)
The patient is extending the finger at the proximal interphalangeal joint against resistance with the metacarpophalangeal joint hyperextended and fixed.

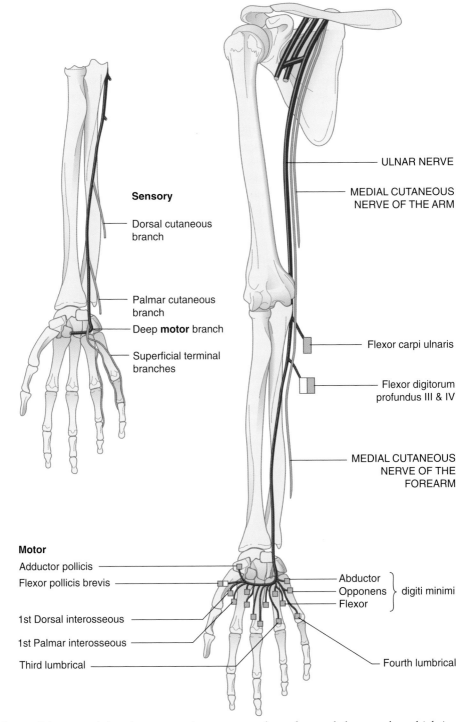

Sensory

Dorsal cutaneous
branch

Palmar cutaneous
branch

Deep **motor** branch

Superficial terminal
branches

ULNAR NERVE

MEDIAL CUTANEOUS
NERVE OF THE ARM

Flexor carpi ulnaris

Flexor digitorum
profundus III & IV

MEDIAL CUTANEOUS
NERVE OF THE
FOREARM

Motor

Adductor pollicis

Flexor pollicis brevis

1st Dorsal interosseous

1st Palmar interosseous

Third lumbrical

Abductor
Opponens ⎬ digiti minimi
Flexor

Fourth lumbrical

Fig. 45 Diagram of the ulnar nerve, its cutaneous branches and the muscles which it
supplies.

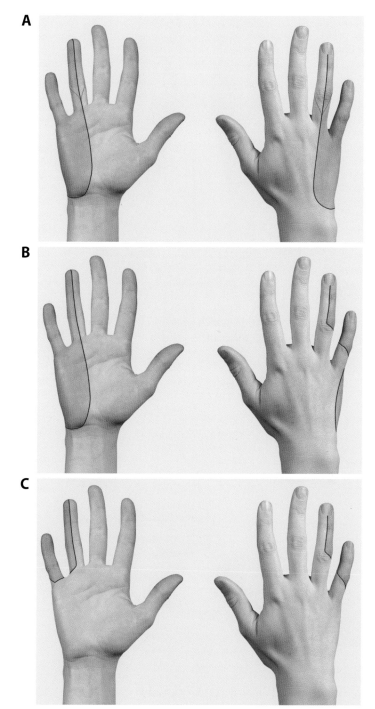

Fig. 46 The approximate areas within which sensory changes may be found in lesions of the ulnar nerve: **A** above the origin of the dorsal cutaneous branch, **B** below the origin of the dorsal cutaneous branch and above the origin of the palmar branch, **C** below the origin of the palmar branch.

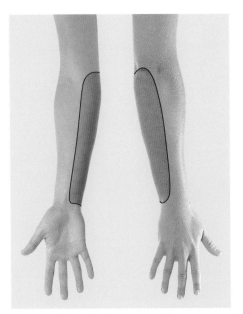

Fig. 47 The approximate area within which sensory changes may be found in lesions of the medial cutaneous nerve of the forearm.

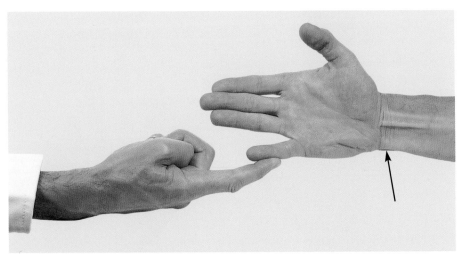

Fig. 48 Flexor Carpi Ulnaris (Ulnar nerve; C7, C8, T1)

The patient is abducting the little finger against resistance. The tendon of flexor carpi ulnaris can be seen and felt (*arrow*) as the muscle comes into action to fix the pisiform bone from which abductor digiti minimi arises. If flexor carpi ulnaris is intact, the tendon is seen even when abductor digiti minimi is paralysed (see also Fig. 49).

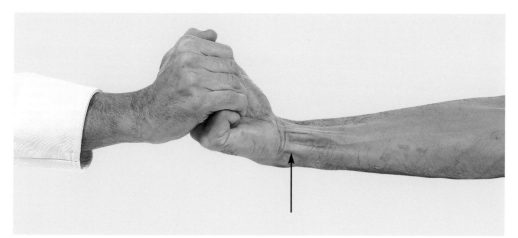

Fig. 49 Flexor Carpi Ulnaris (Ulnar nerve; C7, **C8**, T1)
The patient is flexing and adducting the hand at the wrist against resistance.
Arrow: the tendon can be seen and felt.

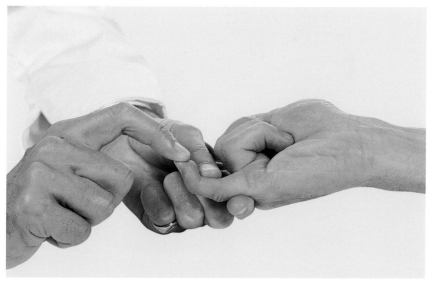

Fig. 50 Flexor Digitorum Profundus III and IV (Ulnar nerve; C7, **C8**)
The patient is flexing the distal interphalangeal joint against resistance while the middle
phalanx is fixed.

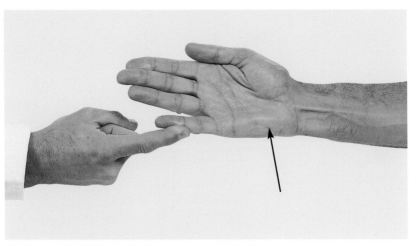

Fig. 51 Abductor Digiti Minimi (Ulnar nerve; **C8, T1**)
The patient is abducting the little finger against resistance.
Arrow: the muscle belly can be felt and seen.

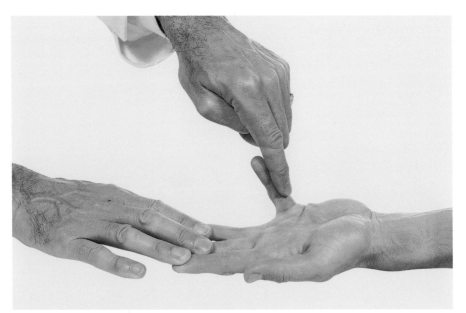

Fig. 52 Flexor Digiti Minimi (Ulnar nerve; **C8, T1**)
The patient is flexing the little finger at the metacarpophalangeal joint against resistance
with the finger extended at both interphalangeal joints.

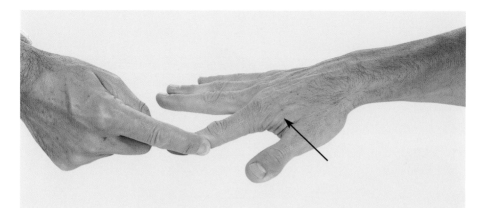

Fig. 53 First Dorsal Interosseous Muscle (Ulnar nerve; C8, **T1**)
The patient is abducting the index finger against resistance.
Arrow: the muscle belly can be felt and usually seen.

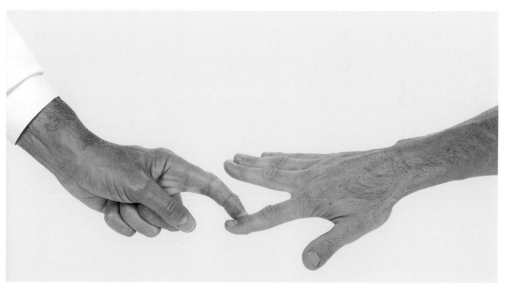

Fig. 54 Second Palmar Interosseous Muscle (Ulnar nerve; C8, **T1**)
The patient is adducting the index finger against resistance.

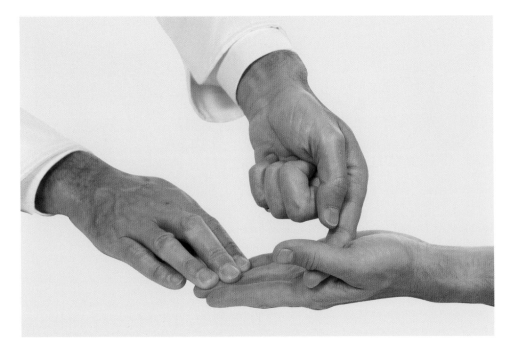

Fig. 55 Adductor Pollicis (Ulnar nerve; C8, **T1**)

The patient is adducting the thumb at right angles to the palm against the resistance of the examiner's finger.

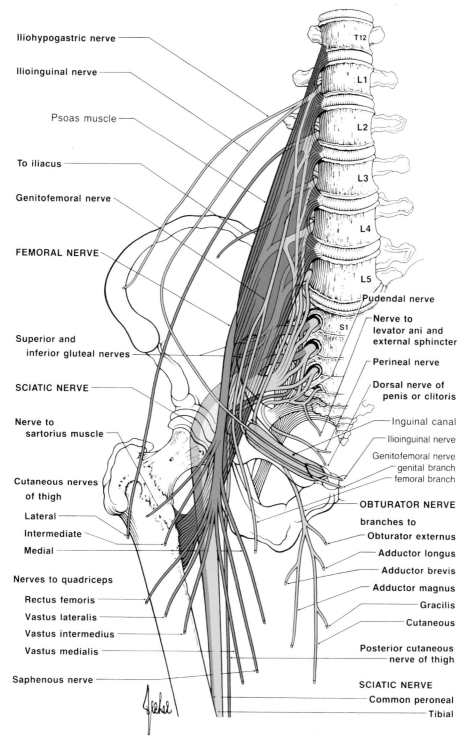

Iliohypogastric nerve

Ilioinguinal nerve

Psoas muscle

To iliacus

Genitofemoral nerve

FEMORAL NERVE

Superior and
inferior gluteal nerves

SCIATIC NERVE

Nerve to
sartorius muscle

Cutaneous nerves
of thigh

Lateral

Intermediate

Medial

Nerves to quadriceps

Rectus femoris

Vastus lateralis

Vastus intermedius

Vastus medialis

Saphenous nerve

T12
L1
L2
L3
L4
L5
S1

Pudendal nerve

Nerve to
levator ani and
external sphincter

Perineal nerve

Dorsal nerve of
penis or clitoris

Inguinal canal

Ilioinguinal nerve

Genitofemoral nerve
genital branch
femoral branch

OBTURATOR NERVE

branches to

Obturator externus

Adductor longus

Adductor brevis

Adductor magnus

Gracilis

Cutaneous

Posterior cutaneous
nerve of thigh

SCIATIC NERVE

Common peroneal

Tibial

Fig. 56 Diagram of the lumbosacral plexus, its branches and the muscles which they supply.

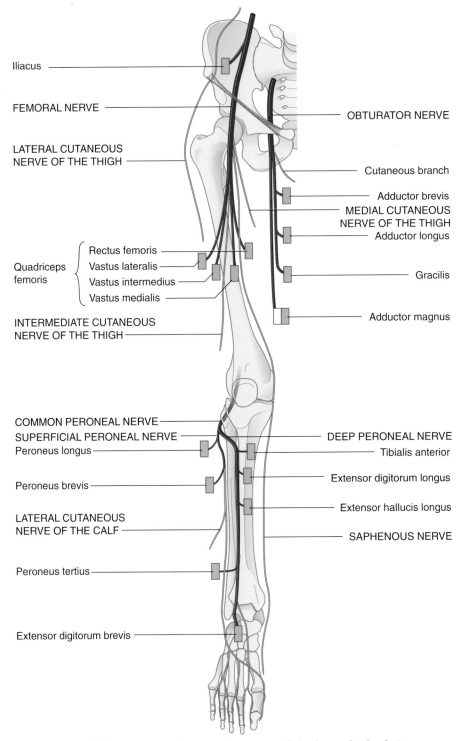

Iliacus

FEMORAL NERVE

LATERAL CUTANEOUS
NERVE OF THE THIGH

OBTURATOR NERVE

Cutaneous branch

Adductor brevis
MEDIAL CUTANEOUS
NERVE OF THE THIGH
Adductor longus

Quadriceps
femoris
{ Rectus femoris
Vastus lateralis
Vastus intermedius
Vastus medialis

Gracilis

INTERMEDIATE CUTANEOUS
NERVE OF THE THIGH

Adductor magnus

COMMON PERONEAL NERVE
SUPERFICIAL PERONEAL NERVE
Peroneus longus

DEEP PERONEAL NERVE
Tibialis anterior

Peroneus brevis

Extensor digitorum longus

Extensor hallucis longus

LATERAL CUTANEOUS
NERVE OF THE CALF

SAPHENOUS NERVE

Peroneus tertius

Extensor digitorum brevis

Fig. 57 Diagram of the nerves on the anterior aspect of the lower limb, their cutaneous branches and the muscles which they supply.

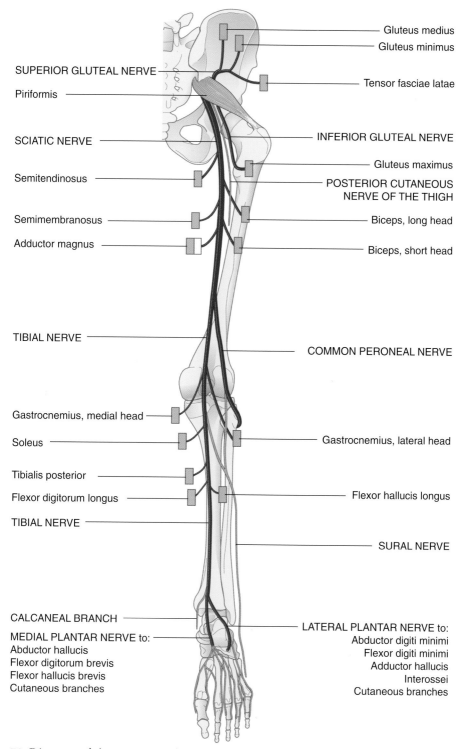

Fig. 58 Diagram of the nerves on the posterior aspect of the lower limb, their cutaneous branches and the muscles which they supply.

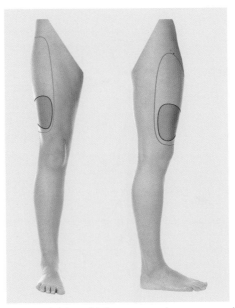

Fig. 59 The approximate area within which sensory changes may be found in lesions of the lateral cutaneous nerve of the thigh.
Usual area shaded, with dark blue line; large area indicated with light blue line.

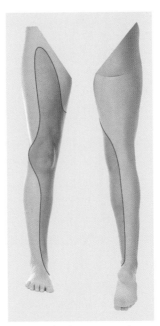

Fig. 60 The approximate area within which sensory changes may be found in lesions of the femoral nerve. (The distribution of the intermediate and medial cutaneous nerves of the thigh and the saphenous nerve.)

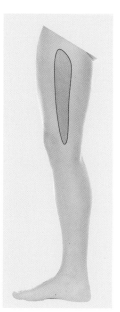

Fig. 61 The approximate area within which sensory changes may be found in lesions of the obturator nerve.

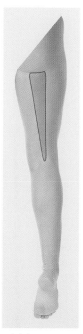

Fig. 62 The approximate area within which sensory changes may be found in lesions of the posterior cutaneous nerve of the thigh.

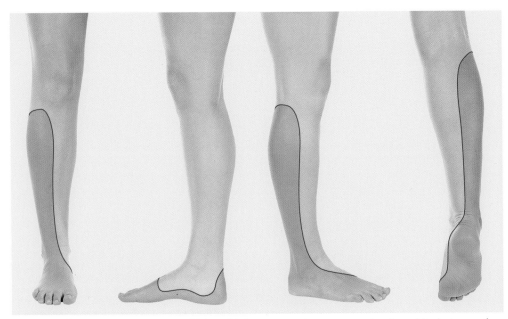

Fig. 63 The approximate area within which sensory changes may be found in lesions of the trunk of the sciatic nerve. (Modified from MRC Special Report No. 54, 1920.)

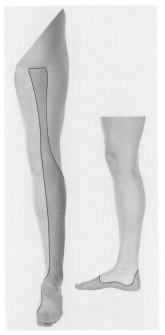

Fig. 64 The approximate area within which sensory changes may be found in lesions of both the sciatic and the posterior cutaneous nerve of the thigh.

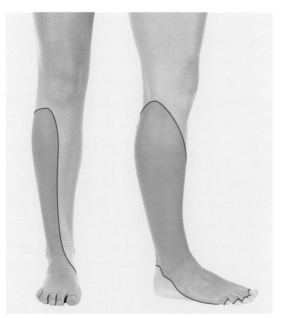

Fig. 65 The approximate area within which sensory changes may be found in lesions of the common peroneal nerve above the origin of the superficial peroneal nerve. (Modified from MRC Special Report No. 54, 1920.)

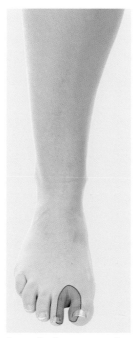

Fig. 66 The approximate area within which sensory changes may be found in lesions of the deep peroneal nerve.

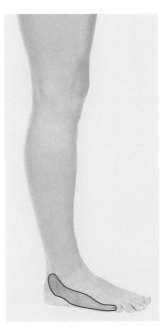

Fig. 67 The approximate area within which sensory changes may be found in lesions of the sural nerve.

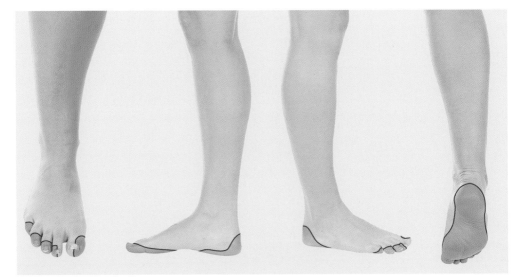

Fig. 68 The approximate area within which sensory changes may be found in lesions of the tibial nerve. (Modified from MRC Special Report No. 54, 1920.)

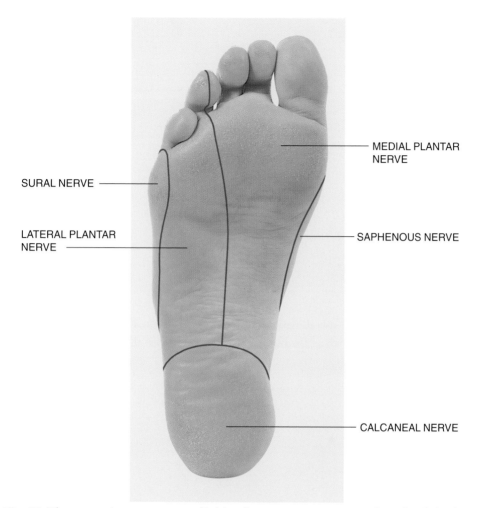

SURAL NERVE

LATERAL PLANTAR
NERVE

MEDIAL PLANTAR
NERVE

SAPHENOUS NERVE

CALCANEAL NERVE

Fig. 69 The approximate areas supplied by the cutaneous nerves to the sole of the foot.

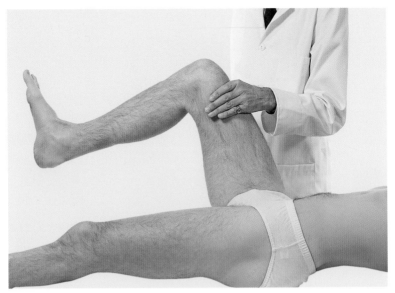

Fig. 70 Iliopsoas
(Branches from L1, 2 and 3 spinal nerves and femoral nerve; **L1, L2**, L3)
The patient is flexing the thigh at the hip against resistance with the leg flexed at the knee and hip.

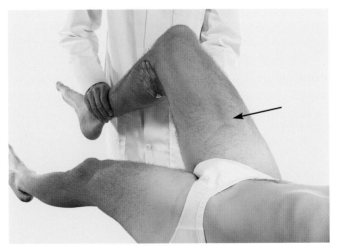

Fig. 71 Quadriceps Femoris (Femoral nerve; L2, **L3, L4**)
The patient is extending the leg against resistance with the limb flexed at the hip and knee. To detect slight weakness, the leg should be fully flexed at the knee.
Arrow: the muscle belly of rectus femoris can be seen and felt.

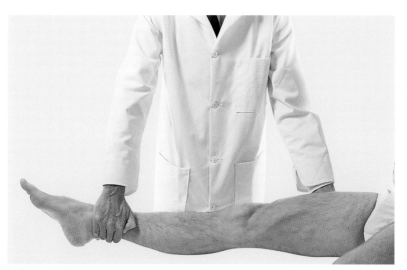

Fig. 72 Adductors (Obturator nerve; **L2, L3, L4**)
The patient lies on his back with the leg extended at the knee, and is adducting the limb against resistance. The muscle bellies can be felt.

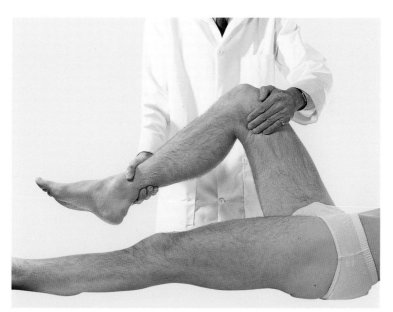

Fig. 73 Gluteus Medius and Minimus (Superior gluteal nerve; **L4, L5, S1**)
The patient lies on his back and is internally rotating the thigh against resistance with the limb flexed at the hip and knee.

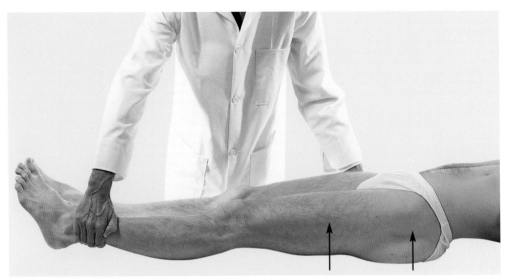

Fig. 74 Gluteus Medius and Minimus and Tensor Fasciae Latae
(Superior gluteal nerve; **L4, L5,** S1)
The patient lies on his back with the leg extended and is abducting the limb against
resistance. *Arrows*: the muscle bellies can be felt and sometimes seen.

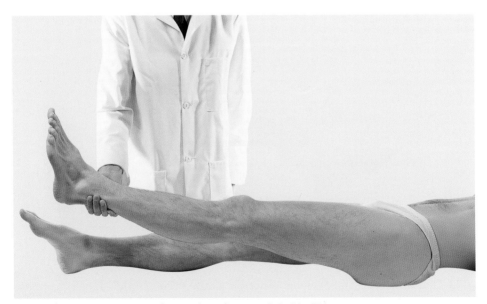

Fig. 75 Gluteus Maximus (Inferior gluteal nerve; L5, **S1,** S2)
The patient lies on his back with the leg extended at the knee and is extending the limb
at the hip against resistance.

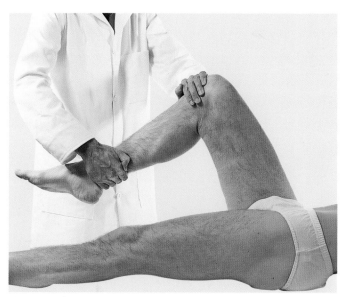

Fig. 76 Hamstring Muscles
(Sciatic nerve. Semitendinosus, semimembranosus and biceps; L5, **S1**, **S2**)
The patient lies on his back with the limb flexed at the hip and knee and is flexing the leg at the knee against resistance.

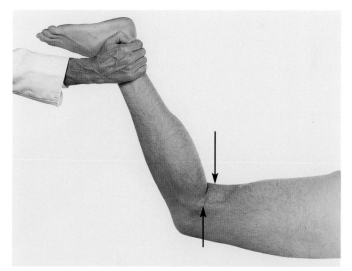

Fig. 77 Hamstring Muscles
(Sciatic nerve. Semitendinosus, semimembranosus and biceps; L5, **S1**, **S2**)
The patient lies on his face and is flexing the leg at the knee against resistance.
Arrows: the tendons of the biceps (laterally) and semitendinosus (medially) can be felt and usually seen.

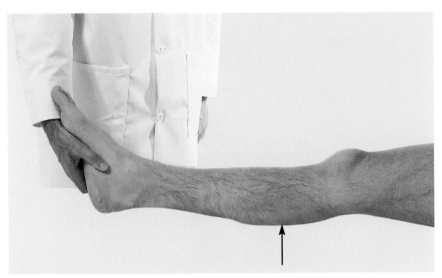

Fig. 78 Gastrocnemius (Tibial nerve; S1, S2)

The patient lies on his back with the leg extended and is plantar-flexing the foot against resistance. *Arrow*: the muscle bellies can be seen and felt. To detect slight weakness, the patient should be asked to stand on one foot, raise the heel from the ground and maintain this position.

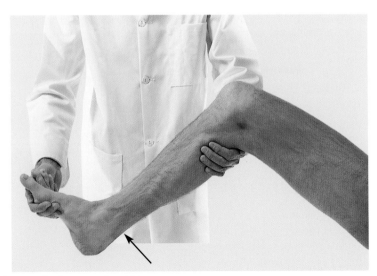

Fig. 79 Soleus (Tibial nerve; S1, S2)

The patient lies on his back with the limb flexed at the hip and knee and is plantar-flexing the foot against resistance. The muscle belly can be felt and sometimes seen. *Arrow*: the Achilles tendon.

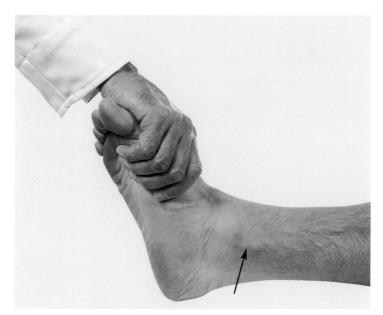

Fig. 80 Tibialis Posterior (Tibial nerve; L4, L5)
The patient is inverting the foot against resistance.
Arrow: the tendon can be seen and felt.

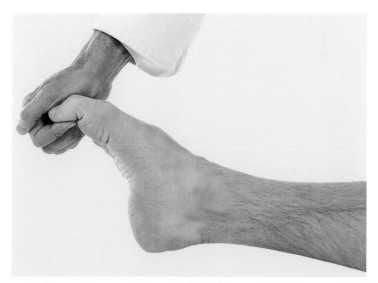

Fig. 81 Flexor Digitorum Longus, Flexor Hallucis Longus (Tibial nerve; L5, S1, S2)
The patient is flexing the toes against resistance.

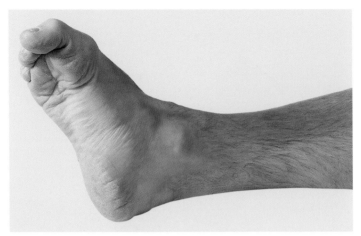

Fig. 82 Small muscles of the foot (medial and lateral plantar nerves; S1, S2)
The patient is cupping the sole of the foot; the small muscles can be felt and sometimes seen.

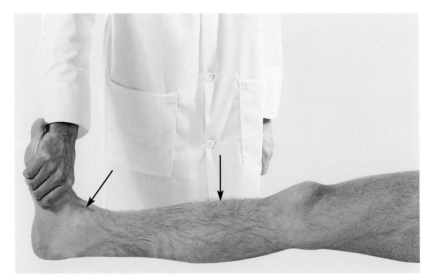

Fig. 83 Tibialis Anterior (Deep peroneal nerve; L4, L5)
The patient is dorsiflexing the foot against resistance.
Arrows: the muscle belly and its tendon can be seen and felt.

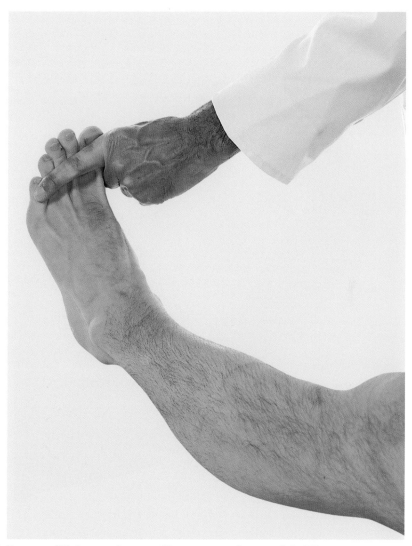

Fig. 84 Extensor Digitorum Longus (Deep peroneal nerve; L5, S1)
The patient is dorsiflexing the toes against resistance. The tendons passing to the lateral four toes can be seen and felt.

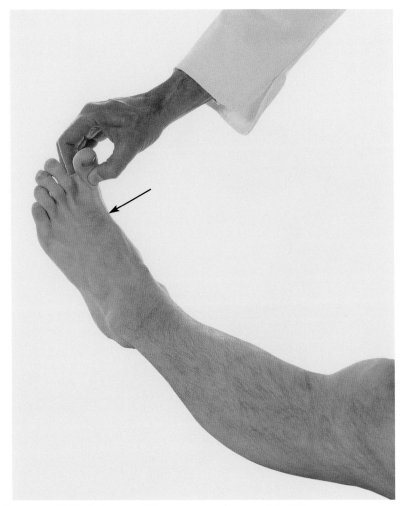

Fig. 85 Extensor Hallucis Longus (Deep peroneal nerve; L5, S1)
The patient is dorsiflexing the distal phalanx of the big toe against resistance.
Arrow: the tendon can be seen and felt.

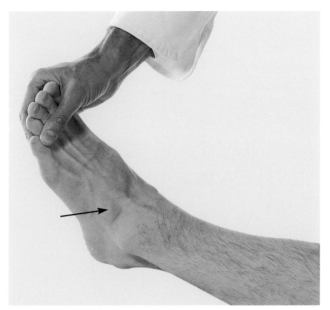

Fig. 86 Extensor Digitorum Brevis (Deep peroneal nerve; L5, S1)
The patient is dorsiflexing the proximal phalanges of the toes against resistance.
Arrow: the muscle belly can be felt and sometimes seen.

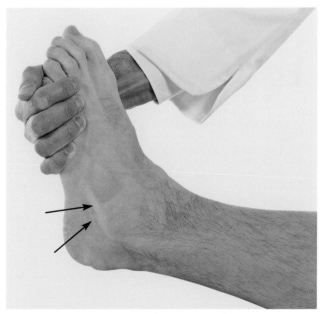

Fig. 87 Peroneus Longus and Brevis (Superficial peroneal nerve; L5, S1)
The patient is everting the foot against resistance. *Upper arrow*: the tendon of peroneus brevis. *Lower arrow*: the tendon of peroneus longus.

DERMATOMES

V₁	1	Supratrochlear nerve	⎤ *Frontal nerve*
	2	Supraorbital nerve	⎦
	3	Lacrimal nerve	
	4	Infratrochlear nerve	⎤ *Nasociliary nerve*
	5	External nasal nerve	⎦
V₂	6	Infraorbital nerve	
	7	Zygomaticofacial nerve	⎤ *Zygomatic nerve*
	8	Zygomaticotemporal nerve	⎦
V₃	9	Auriculotemporal nerve	
	10	Buccal nerve	
	11	Mental nerve	
C2	12	Greater auricular nerve	
	13	Lesser occipital nerve	
	14	Greater occipital nerve	
C3	15	Transverse cervical nerve	
	16	C3 dorsal ramus	
C4	17	C4 dorsal ramus	

Figs 88, 89, 90 The approximate areas within which sensory changes may be found in lesions of the trigeminal nerve and its branches.

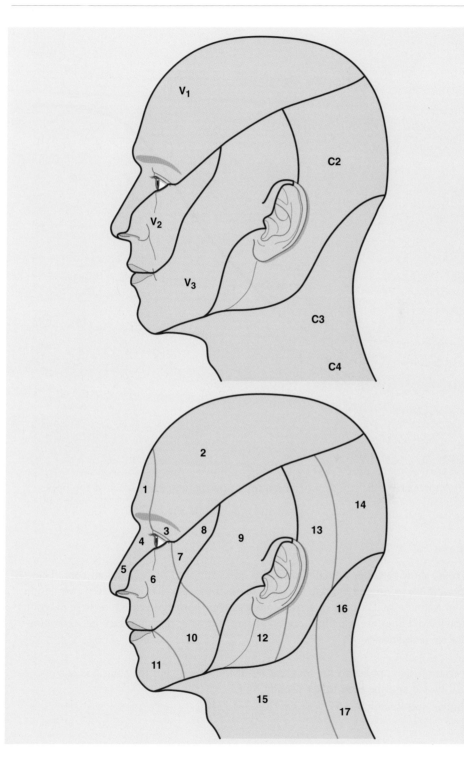

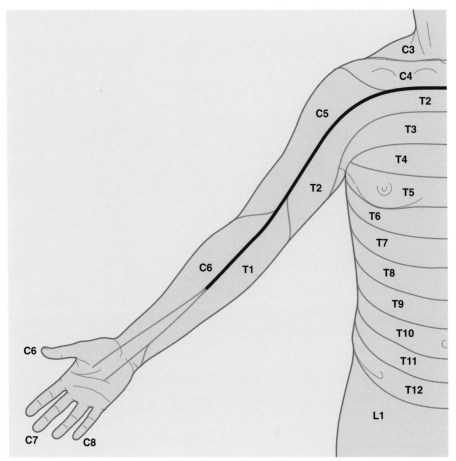

Fig. 91 Approximate distribution of dermatomes on the anterior aspect of the upper limb.

Figs 91–94 show the approximate cutaneous areas supplied by each spinal root. There is considerable variation and overlap between dermatomes, so that an isolated root lesion results in a much smaller area of sensory impairment than is indicated in these diagrams. The heavy axial lines are usually more consistent, showing the boundary between non-consecutive dermatomes.

This variation also applies to the innervation of the fingers, but the thumb is usually supplied by C6 and the little finger usually by C8.
(See Inouye and Buchthal (1977) *Brain* **100**: 731–748.)

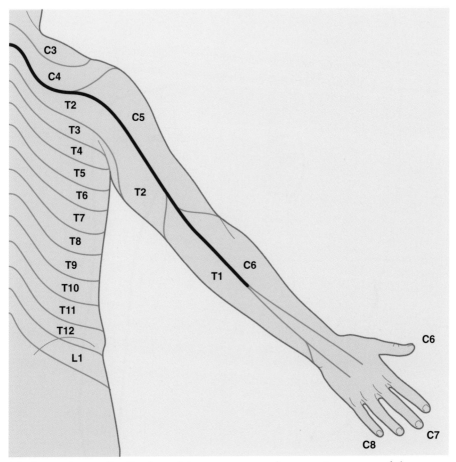

Fig. 92 Approximate distribution of dermatomes on the posterior aspect of the upper limb.

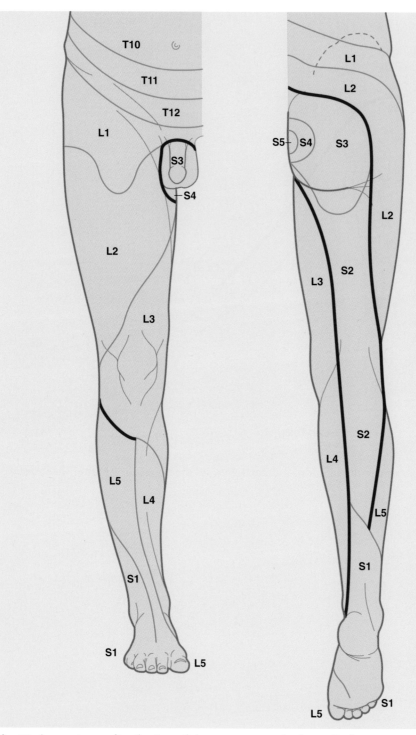

Fig. 93 Approximate distribution of dermatomes on the lower limb.

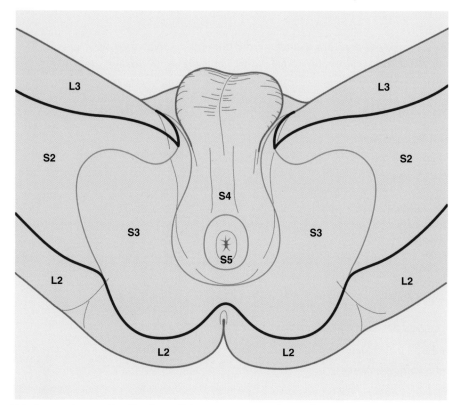

Fig. 94 Approximate distribution of dermatomes on the perineum.

NERVE AND MAIN ROOT SUPPLY OF MUSCLES

The list given below does not include all the muscles innervated by these nerves, but only those more commonly tested, either clinically or electrically, and shows the order of innervation.

Upper Limb	Spinal Roots
Spinal Accessory Nerve	
Trapezius	C3, C4
Brachial Plexus	
Rhomboids	C4, C5
Serratus anterior	C5, C6, C7
Pectoralis major	
Clavicular	C5, C6
Sternal	C6, **C7**, C8
Supraspinatus	C5, C6
Infraspinatus	C5, C6
Latissimus dorsi	C6, **C7**, C8
Teres major	C5, C6, C7
Axillary Nerve	
Deltoid	**C5**, C6
Musculocutaneous Nerve	
Biceps	C5, C6
Brachialis	C5, C6
Radial Nerve	
Triceps { Long head / Lateral head / Medial head }	C6, **C7**, C8
Brachioradialis	C5, **C6**
Extensor carpi radialis longus	C5, **C6**
Posterior Interosseous Nerve	
Supinator	C6, C7
Extensor carpi ulnaris	C7, C8
Extensor digitorum	C7, C8
Abductor pollicis longus	C7, C8
Extensor pollicis longus	C7, C8
Extensor pollicis brevis	C7, C8
Extensor indicis	C7, C8
Median Nerve	
Pronator teres	C6, C7
Flexor carpi radialis	C6, C7
Flexor digitorum superficialis	C7, **C8**, T1
Abductor pollicis brevis	C8, **T1**
Flexor pollicis brevis*	C8, **T1**
Opponens pollicis	C8, **T1**
Lumbricals I & II	C8, **T1**

COMMONLY TESTED MOVEMENTS

Movement	UMN	Root	Reflex	Nerve	Muscle
Upper Limb					
Shoulder abduction	++	C5		Axillary	Deltoid
Elbow flexion		C5.6	+	Musculocutaneuos	Biceps
		C6	+	Radial	Brachioradialis
Elbow extension	+	C7	+	Radial	Triceps
Radial wrist extension	+	C6		Radial	Extensor carpi radialis longus
Finger extension	+	C7		Posterior interosseus	Extensor digitorum communis
Finger flexion		C8	+	Anterior interosseus	Flexor pollicis longus
					Flexor digitorum profundus (index finger)
				Median	All other flexors
				Ulnar	Flexor digitorum profundus (ring & little fingers)
Finger abduction	++	T1		Ulnar	First dorsal interosseus
				Median	Abductor pollicis brevis
Lower Limb					
Hip flexion	++	L1.2			Iliopsoas
Hip adduction		L2.3	+	Obturator	Adductors
Hip extension		L5.S1		Sciatic	Gluteus maximus
Knee flexion	+	S1		Sciatic	Hamstrings
Knee extension		L3.4	+	Femoral	Quadriceps
Ankle dorsiflexion	++	L4		Deep peroneal	Tibialis anterior
Ankle eversion		L5.S1		Superficial peroneal	Peronei
Ankle plantarflexion		S1.S2	+	Tibial	Gastrocnemius, Soleus
Big toe extension		L5		Deep peroneal	Extensor hallucis longus

The table shows some commonly tested movements, the principal muscle involved with its roots and nerve supply. The column headed UMN indicates those movements which are preferentially weak in upper motor neuron lesions.

Anterior Interosseous Nerve

Pronator quadratus	C7, **C8**
Flexor digitorum profundus I & II	C7, **C8**
Flexor pollicis longus	C7, **C8**

Ulnar Nerve

Flexor carpi ulnaris	C7, **C8**, T1
Flexor digitorum profundus III & IV	C7, **C8**
Hypothenar muscles	**C8, T1**
Adductor pollicis	**C8, T1**
Flexor pollicis brevis	**C8, T1**
Palmar interossei	**C8, T1**
Dorsal interossei	**C8, T1**
Lumbricals III & IV	**C8, T1**

Lower Limb — Spinal Roots

Femoral Nerve

Iliopsoas		L1, **L2**, L3
Rectus femoris	⎫	
Vastus lateralis	⎪	
Vastus intermedius	⎬ Quadriceps femoris	L2, **L3, L4**
Vastus medialis	⎭	

Obturator Nerve

Adductor longus	⎫	
Adductor magnus	⎬	L2, **L3, L4**

Superior Gluteal Nerve

Gluteus medus and minimus	⎫	
Tensor fasciae latae	⎬	**L4, L5**, S1

Inferior Gluteal Nerve

Gluteus maximus	**L5, S1**, S2

Sciatic and Tibial Nerves

Semitendinosus		L5, **S1, S2**
Biceps		L5, **S1, S2**
Semimembranosus		L5, **S1, S2**
Gastrocnemius and soleus		**S1, S2**
Tibialis posterior		**L4, L5**
Flexor digitorum longus		L5, **S1, S2**
Abductor hallucis		
Abductor digiti minimi	⎫ Small muscles of foot	**S1, S2**
Interossei	⎭	

Sciatic and Common Peroneal Nerves

Tibialis anterior	**L4, L5**
Extensor digitorum longus	**L5, S1**
Extensor hallucis longus	**L5, S1**
Extensor digitorum brevis	**L5, S1**
Peroneus longus	**L5, S1**
Peroneus brevis	**L5, S1**

Flexor pollicis brevis is often supplied wholly or partially by the ulnar nerve.